RENAL DIET COOKBOOK

40+ Recipes: Meat and Vegetable

How to Take Control of Your Kidney Disease and Avoid Dialysis.

Irene Simmons

Table of Contents

Introduction

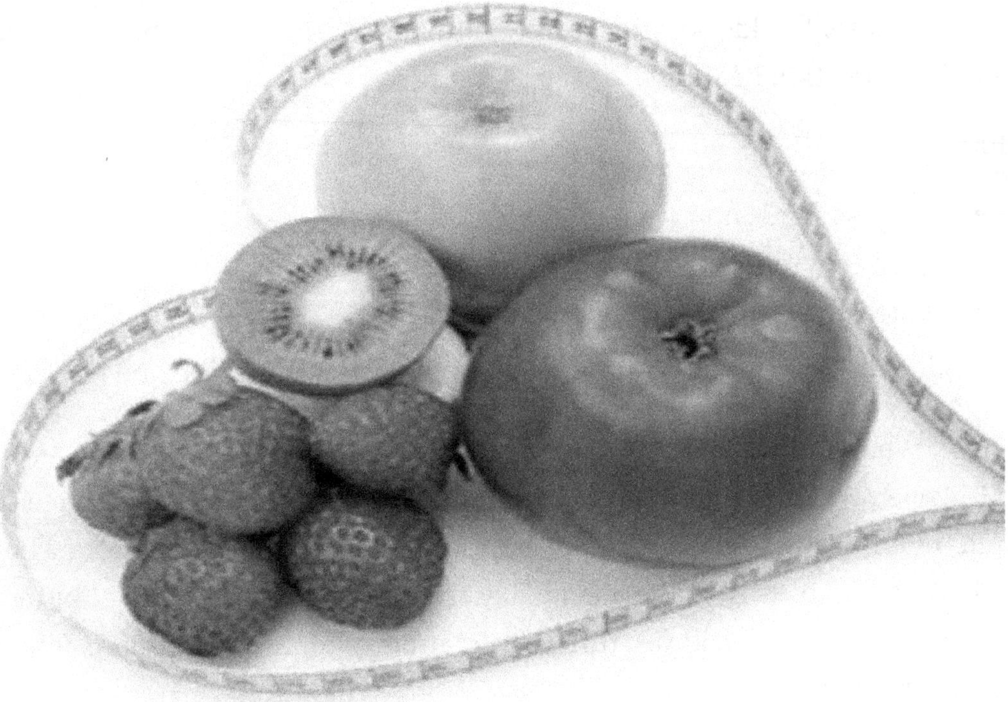

Human health hangs in a complete balance when all of its interconnected bodily mechanisms function properly in perfect sync. Without its major organs working normally, the body soon suffers indelible damage. Kidney malfunction is one such example, and it is not just the entire water balance that is disturbed by the kidney disease, but a number of other diseases also emerge due to this problem. Kidney diseases are progressive in nature, meaning that if left unchecked and uncontrolled, they can ultimately lead to permanent kidney damage. That is why it is essential to control and manage the disease and put a halt to its progress, which can be done through medicinal and natural means. While medicines can guarantee only thirty percent of the cure, a change of lifestyle and diet can prove to be miraculous with seventy percent of guaranteed results. A kidney-friendly diet and lifestyle not only saves the kidneys from excess minerals but they also aid medicines to work actively. Treatment without a good diet, hence, proves to be useless. In this renal diet cookbook, we shall bring out the basic facts about kidney diseases, their symptoms, causes, and diagnosis. This preliminary introduction can help the readers understand the problem clearly; then, we shall discuss the role of renal diet and kidney-friendly lifestyle in curbing the diseases. And it's not just that. The book also contains a range of delicious renal diet recipes that will guarantee luscious flavors and good health.

Despite their tiny size, the kidneys perform a number of functions, which are vital for the body to be able to function healthily.

These include:

- Filtering excess fluids and waste from the blood
- Creating the enzyme known as renin, which regulates blood pressure,
- Ensuring bone marrow creates red blood cells,
- Controlling calcium and phosphorus levels through absorption and excretion.

Unfortunately, when kidney disease reaches a chronic stage, these functions start to stop working. However, with the right treatment and lifestyle, it is possible to manage symptoms and continue living well. This is even more applicable in the earlier stages of the disease. Tactlessly, 10% of all adults over the age of 20 will experience some form of kidney disease in their lifetime. There are a variety of different treatments for kidney disease, which depend on the cause of the disease.

Kidney (or renal) diseases are affecting around 14% of the adult population, according to international stats. In the US, approx. 661.000 Americans suffer from kidney dysfunction. Out of these patients, 468.000 proceed to dialysis treatment, and the rest have one active kidney transplant.

The high quantities of diabetes and heart illness are additionally related to kidney dysfunction, and sometimes one condition, for example, diabetes, may prompt the other.

With such a significant number of high rates, possibly the best course of treatment is the contravention of dialysis, which makes people depend upon clinical and crisis facility meds on any occasion multiple times every week. In this manner, if your kidney has just given a few indications of brokenness, you can forestall dialysis through an eating routine, something that we will talk about in this book.

What to Know About the Kidney Disease

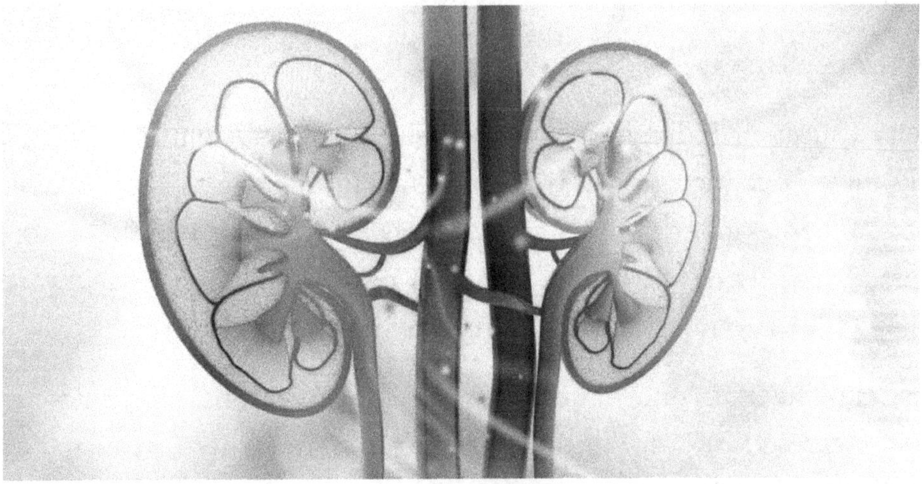

Kidney disease is becoming more prevalent in the United States, and so we need to learn as much about it as we can. The more we educate ourselves, the more we can do to take care of this important bodily system. If you've been diagnosed with chronic kidney disease (CKD), education can empower you to most effectively and purposefully manage the disease. Once you have a full understanding of what chronic kidney disease is, you can begin to take charge of your evolving health needs. Making healthy changes early in the stages of kidney disease will help determine how well you will manage your kidney health. I am here to guide you, every step of the way. Like any new process, it may seem intimidating at first. But this chapter provides the foundation for learning, and will help you understand kidney disease as you begin your journey to healthier kidneys.

What Do the Kidneys Do?

Our kidneys are small, but they do powerful things to keep our body in balance. They are bean-shaped, about the size of a fist, and are located in the middle of the back, on the left and right sides of the spine, just below the rib cage. When everything is working properly, the kidneys do many important jobs such as:

- Filter waste materials from the blood

- Remove extra fluid, or water, from the body
- Release hormones that help manage blood pressure
- Stimulate bone marrow to make red blood cells
- Make an active form of vitamin D that promotes strong, healthy bones

What Causes Kidney Disease?

There are many causes of kidney disease, including physical injury or disorders that can damage the kidneys, but the two leading causes of kidney disease are diabetes and high blood pressure. These underlying conditions also put people at risk for developing cardiovascular disease. Early treatment may not only slow down the progression of the disease, but also reduce your risk of developing heart disease or stroke.

Kidney disease can affect anyone, at any age. African Americans, Hispanics, and American Indians are at increased risk for kidney failure, because these groups have a greater prevalence of diabetes and high blood pressure.

When we digest protein, our bodies create waste products. As blood flows through the capillaries, the waste products are filtered through the urine. Substances such as protein and red blood cells are too big to pass through the capillaries and so stay in the blood. All the extra work takes a toll on the kidneys. When kidney disease is detected in the early stages, several treatments may prevent the worsening of the disease. If kidney disease is detected in the later stages, high amounts of protein in your urine, called macro albuminuria, can lead to end-stage renal disease.

The second leading cause of kidney disease is high blood pressure, also known as hypertension. One in three Americans is at risk for kidney disease because of hypertension. Although there is no cure for hypertension, certain medications, a low-sodium diet, and physical activity can lower blood pressure.

The kidneys help manage blood pressure, but when blood pressure is high, the heart has to work overtime at pumping blood. When the force of blood flow is high, blood vessels start to stretch so the blood can flow more easily. The stretching and scarring weakens the blood vessels throughout the entire body, including the kidneys. And when the kidneys' blood vessels are injured, they may not remove the waste and extra fluid from the body, creating a dangerous cycle, because the extra fluid in the blood vessels can increase blood pressure even more.

With diabetes, excess blood sugar remains in the bloodstream. The high blood sugar levels can damage the blood vessels in the kidneys and elsewhere in the body. And since high blood pressure is a complication from diabetes, the extra pressure can weaken the walls of the blood vessels, which can lead to a heart attack or stroke.

Other conditions, such as drug abuse and certain autoimmune diseases, can also cause injury to the kidneys. In fact, every drug we put into our body has to pass through the kidneys for filtration.

An autoimmune disease is one in which the immune system, designed to protect the body from illness, sees the body as an invader and attacks its own systems, including the kidneys. Some forms of lupus, for example, attack the kidneys. Another autoimmune disease that can lead to kidney failure is Good pasture syndrome, a group of conditions that affect the kidneys and the lungs. The damage to the kidneys from autoimmune diseases can lead to chronic kidney disease and kidney failure.

Treatment Plans for Chronic Kidney Disease (Cod)

The best way to manage CKD is to be an active participant in your treatment program, regardless of your stage of renal disease. Proper treatment involves a combination of working with a healthcare team, adhering to a renal diet, and making healthy lifestyle decisions. These can all have a profoundly positive effect on your kidney disease—especially watching how you eat.

Working with your healthcare team. When you have kidney disease, working in partnership with your healthcare team can be extremely important in your treatment program as well as being personally empowering. Regularly meeting with your physician or healthcare team can arm you with resources and information that help you make informed decisions regarding your treatment needs, and provide you with a much needed opportunity to vent, share information, get advice, and receive support in effectively managing this illness.

Adhering to a renal diet. The heart of this book is the renal diet. Sticking to this diet can make a huge difference in your health and vitality. Like any change, following the diet may not be easy at first. Important changes to your diet, particularly early on, can possibly prevent the need for dialysis. These changes include limiting salt, eating a low-protein diet, reducing fat intake, and getting enough calories if you need to lose weight. Be honest with yourself first and foremost—learn what you need, and consider your personal goals and obstacles. Start by making small changes. It is okay to have some slip-ups—we all do. With guidance and support, these small changes will become habits of your promising new lifestyle. In no time, you will begin taking control of your diet and health.

Making healthy lifestyle decisions. Lifestyle choices play a crucial part in our health, especially when it comes to helping regulate kidney disease. Lifestyle choices such as allotting time for physical activity, getting enough sleep, managing weight, reducing stress, and limiting smoking and alcohol will help you take control of your overall health, making it easier to manage your kidney disease. Follow this simple formula: Keep toxins out of your body as much as you can, and build up your immune system with a good balance of exercise, relaxation, and sleep.

What to do to Slow down Kidney Disease

A kidney disease diagnosis can seem devastating at first. The news may come as a shock for some people, who may not have experienced any symptoms. It's important to remember that you can control your progress and improvement through diet and lifestyle changes, even when a prognosis is serious. Taking steps to improve your health can make a significant effort to slow the progression of kidney disease and improve your quality of life.

Focus on Weight Loss

Losing weight is one of the most common reasons for going on a diet. It's also one of the best ways to treat kidney disease and prevent further damage. Carrying excess weight contributes to high toxicity levels in the body, by storing toxins instead of releasing them through the kidneys. Eating foods high in trans fats, sugar, and excess sodium contribute to obesity, which affects close to one third of North Americans and continues to rise in many other countries, where fast foods are becoming easier to access and less expensive. Losing weight is a difficult cycle for many, who often diet temporarily only to return to unhealthy habits after reaching a milestone, which results in gaining the weight back, thus causing an unhealthy "yo-yo" diet effect.

There are some basic and easy changes you can make to shed those first pounds, which will begin to take the pressure off the kidneys and help you onto the path of regular weight loss:

Drink plenty of water. If you can't drink eight glasses a day, try adding unsweetened natural sparkling water or herbal teas to increase your water intake.

Reduce the amount of sugar and carbohydrates you consume. This doesn't require adapting to a ketogenic or low-carb diet – you'll notice a major change after ditching soda and reducing the bread and pasta by half.

Take your time to eat and avoid rushing. If you need to eat in a hurry, grab a piece of fruit or a small portion of macadamia nuts. Avoid sugary and salty foods as much as possible. Choose fresh fruits over potato chips and chocolate bars.

Create a short list of kidney-friendly foods that you enjoy and use this as your reference or guide when grocery shopping. This will help you stock up on snacks, ingredients, and foods for your kitchen that work well within your renal diet plan, at the same time reducing your chances of succumbing to the temptation of eating a bag of salted pretzels or chocolate.

Once you make take a few steps towards changing the way you eat, it will get easier. Making small changes at first is the key to success and to progressing with a new way of eating and living. If you are already in the habit of consuming packaged foods - such as crackers, chips, processed dips, sauces and sodas, for example - try cutting down on one or two items at a time, and over a while, gradually eliminate and cut down other items. Slowly replace these with fresh foods and healthier choices, so that your body has a chance to adapt without extreme cravings that often occur during sudden changes.

Quit Smoking and Reduce Alcohol

It's not easy to quit smoking or using recreational drugs, especially where there has been long-term use and the effects have already made an impact on your health. At some point, you'll begin to notice a difference in the way you feel and how your body changes over time. This includes chronic coughing related to respiratory conditions, shortness of breath, and a lack of energy. These changes may be subtle at first, and it may appear as though there is minimal damage or none at all, though smoking inevitably catches up with age and contributes to the development of cancer, premature aging and kidney damage. The more toxins we consume or add to our body, the more challenging it becomes for the kidneys to work efficiently, which eventually slows their ability to function.

For most people, quitting "cold turkey" or all at once is not an option, because of the withdrawal symptoms and increased chances of starting again. This method, however, can work if applied with a strong support system and a lot of determination, though it's not the best option for everyone. Reducing smoking on your own, or switching to e-cigarettes or a patch or medication, can help significantly over time. Setting goals of reduction until the point of quitting can be a beneficial way to visualize success and provide a sense of motivation. The following tips may also be useful for quitting smoking and other habit-forming substances:

Join a support group and talk to other people who relate to you. Share your struggles, ideas, and thoughts, which will help others as well as yourself during this process.

Track your progress on a calendar or in a notebook, either by pen and paper or on an application. This can serve as a motivator, as well as a means to display how you've done so far and where you can improve. For example, you may have reduced your smoking from ten to seven cigarettes per day, then increased to nine. This may indicate a slight change that can keep in mind to focus on reducing your intake further, from nine cigarettes to seven or six per day, and so on.

Be aware of stressors in your life that cause you to smoke or use substances. If these factors are avoidable, make every effort to minimize or stop them from impacting your life. This may include specific people, places, or situations that can "trigger" a craving or make you feel more likely to use than usual. If there are situations that you cannot avoid, such as family, work, or school-related situations, consult with a trusted friend or someone you can confide in who can be present with you during these instances.

Don't be afraid to ask for help. Many people cannot quit on their own without at least some assistance from others. Seeking the guidance and expertise of a counselor or medical professional to better yourself can be one of the most important decisions you make to improve the quality of your life.

Getting Active

One of the most important ways to keep fit and healthy is by staying active and engaging in regular exercise. Regular movement is key, and exercise is different for everyone, depending on their abilities and options available. Fortunately, there are unlimited ways to customize an exercise routine or plan that can suit any lifestyle, perhaps low impact to start, or if you're ready, engage in a more vigorous workout. For many people experiencing kidney disease, one of the major struggles is losing weight and living a sedentary life, where movement is generally minimal and exercise is generally not practiced. Smoking, eating processed foods, and not getting the required nutrition can further impair the body in such a way that exercise is seen as a hurdle and a challenge that is best avoided. Making lifestyle changes is not something that should be done all at once, but over a while - especially during the early stages of renal disease - so that the impact of the condition is minimized over time and becomes more manageable.

Where can you begin, if you haven't exercised at all or for a long period? For starters, don't sign up for a marathon or engage in any strenuous activities unless it is safe to do so. Start slow and take your time. Before taking on any new movements - whether it is minimal, low-impact walking or stretching, or a more moderate to the high-impact regimen - always talk to your doctor to rule out any impact this may have on other existing conditions, such as blood pressure and respiratory conditions, as well as your kidneys. Most, if not all, physicians will likely recommend exercise as part of the treatment plan but may advise beginning slowly if your body isn't used to exercise.

Simple techniques to introduce exercise into your life require a commitment. This can begin with a quick 15-minute walk or jog and a 10-or 15-minute stretch in the morning before starting your day. There are several easy, introductory techniques to consider, including the following:

Take a walk for 10 to 15 minutes each day, at least three or four days each week. If you find it difficult at first, due to cramping, respiratory issues, or other conditions, walk slowly and breathe deeply. Make sure you feel relaxed during your walks. Find a scenic path or area in your neighborhood that is pleasant and gives you something to enjoy, such as a beautiful sunset or forested park. Bring a bottle of water to keep yourself hydrated.

Stretch for five minutes once a day. This doesn't mean you need to do any intricate yoga poses or specific techniques. Moving your ankles, wrists, and arms in circles and standing every so often (if you sit often) and twisting your torso can help release stress and improve your blood flow, which lowers blood pressure and helps your body transport nutrients to areas in need of repair.

Practice breathing long, measured breaths. This will help prepare you for more endurance-based exercise, such as jogging, long walks, cycling, and swimming. Count to five on each inhale and exhale, and practice moving slowly as you breathe, to "sync" or coordinate your body's movements with your breathing. If you have difficulty with the respiratory system, take it slow and don't push yourself. If you feel weak or out of breath, stop immediately and try again later or the next day at a slower pace.

Start a beginner's yoga class and learn the fundamentals of various poses and stretches. It is helpful to arrive early and speak with the instructor, who can provide guidance on which modifications work best if needed. They may also be able to provide tips on how to approach certain poses or movements that can be challenging for beginners so that you feel more comfortable and knowledgeable before you start.

If you smoke, exercise will present more of a challenge on your lungs and respiratory function. Once you become accustomed to a beginner's level and become moderately active, you may notice it takes more effort, which requires an increase in lung capacity and oxygen. Smoking will eventually present a challenge, and where quitting can be a long-term and difficult goal in itself, make an effort to cut back as much as it takes to allow your body's movements and exercise continue. In time, you may find quitting becomes easier and more achievable than expected!

Once you get into a basic routine, there is a wide variety of individual and team activities to consider for your life. If you are a social person, joining a baseball team or badminton club

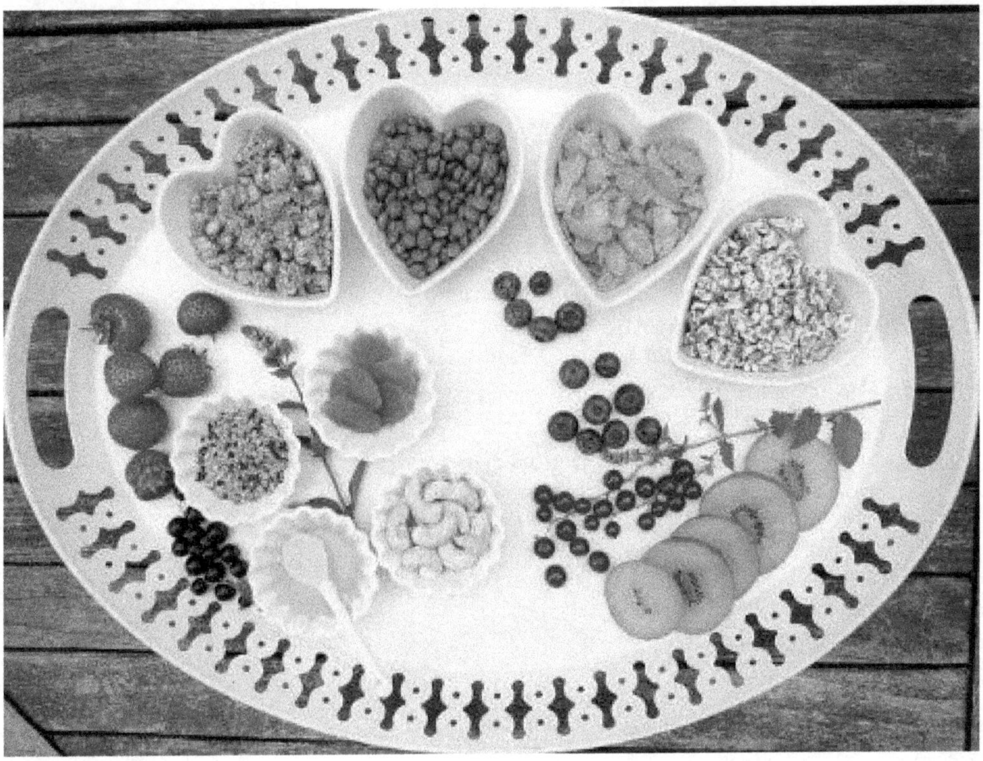

may be ideal. For more solitary options, consider swimming, cycling, or jogging. Many gyms and community centers provide monthly plans and may offer a free trial period to see if their facilities work for you. This is a great opportunity to try new classes and equipment to gauge how much you can achieve, even if in the early stages of exercise so that you can decide whether to pursue dance aerobics, spin classes and/or weight training. Some gyms will provide a free consultation with a personal trainer to set a simple plan towards weight loss and strength training goals.

Symptoms of kidney disease?

If kidney disease progresses, then the blood level of end products of metabolism increases; this in turn, is the cause of feeling unwell. Various health problems may occur, such as high blood pressure, anemia (anemia), bone disease, premature cardiovascular calcification, discoloration, and change in the composition and volume of urine.

As the disease progresses, the main symptoms can be:

- Weakness, a feeling of weakness
- Trouble sleeping
- Lack of appetite
- Dry skin, itchy skin
- Muscle cramps especially at night
- Swelling in the legs
- Swelling around the eyes, especially in the morning

The Causes of Kidney Failure

Renal disease, according to experts, requires early diagnosis and targeted treatment to prevent or delay both a condition of acute or chronic renal failure and the appearance of cardiovascular complications to which it is often associated.

In fact, hypertension and diabetes, not adequately controlled by drug therapy, prostatic hypertrophy, kidney stones or bulky tumors can promote onset as they reduce the normal flow of urine, increase the pressure inside the kidneys and limit functionality.

Or the kidney damage can be determined by inflammatory processes (pyelonephritis, glomerulonephritis) or by the formation of cysts inside the kidneys (polycystic kidney disease) or by the chronic use of some drugs, alcohol and drugs consumed in excess.

A fundamental role in alleviating the work of the already compromised kidneys is carried out by the diet which is, therefore, the first prevention. It must be studied with an expert nutritionist or a nephrologist in order to maintain or reach an ideal weight on the one hand and on the other to reduce the intake of sodium (salt), and the consequent control of blood pressure, and / or other substances (minerals), without creating malnutrition or nutritional deficiencies. Particular attention should also be paid to cholesterol, triglycerides and blood sugar levels.

Understanding what causes kidney failure goes a long way to deciding just what kind of treatment you should focus on. The most important factor that you should focus on is, of course, your diet. But as you focus on your diet, make sure that you are following your doctor's instructions, in the event of other complications. Let us look at a few of the common causes of kidney diseases.

Diabetes

We do know that diabetes is one of the leading causes of CKD. But we have yet to understand in detail why and how it can cause so much harm to the kidneys.

Time for a crash course in diabetes. What many may already know is that diabetes affects our body's insulin production rate. But what many may not know is the extent of damage that diabetes can cause to the kidneys.

High Blood Pressure

An important thing to remember here is that high blood pressure can be both a cause and symptom of CKD, similar to the case of diabetes.

So, what exactly is blood pressure? People often throw the term around, but they are unable to pinpoint exactly what happens when the pressure in the blood increases.

Autoimmune Diseases

IgA nephropathy and lupus are two examples of autoimmune diseases that can lead to kidney diseases. But just what exactly are autoimmune diseases?

They are conditions where your immune system perceives your body as a threat and begins to attack it.

We all know that the immune system is like the defense force of our body. It is responsible for guiding the soldiers of our body, known as white blood cells, or WBCs. The immune system is responsible for fighting against foreign materials, such as viruses and bacteria. When the system senses these foreign bodies, various fighter cells, including the WBCs, are deployed in order to combat the threat.

Typically, your immune system is a self-learning system. This means that it is capable of understanding the threat and memorizing its features, behaviors, and attack patterns. This is an important capability of the immune system since it allows the system to differentiate between our own cells and foreign cells. But when you have an autoimmune disease, your immune system suddenly considers certain parts of your body, such as your skin or joints, as foreign. It then proceeds to create antibodies that begin to

Diagnosis

There are two simple tests that your family doctor can prescribe to diagnose a kidney disease.

Blood test: glomerular filtration rate (GFR) and serum creatinine level. Creatinine is one of those end products of protein metabolism, the level of which in the blood depends on age, gender, muscle mass, nutrition, physical activity, the foods taken before taking the sample (for example, a lot of meat was eaten), and some drugs. Creatinine is removed from the body through the kidneys, and if the work of the kidneys slows down, the level of creatinine in the blood plasma increases. Determining the level of creatinine alone is not sufficient for the diagnosis of chronic kidney disease since its value begins to exceed the upper limit of the norm only when GFR is decreased by half. GFR is calculated using a formula that includes four parameters which are; the creatinine reading, age, gender, and race of the patient. GFR shows the level at which the kidneys can filter. In the case of chronic kidney disease, the GFR indicator indicates the stage of the severity of kidney disease.

Urine analysis: the content of albumin in the urine is determined; also, the values of albumin and creatinine in the urine are determined by each other. Albumin is a protein in the urine that usually enters the urine in minimal quantities. Even a small increase in the level of albumin in the urine in some people may be an early sign of incipient kidney disease, especially in those with diabetes and high blood pressure. In the case of normal kidney function, albumin in the urine should not be more than 3 mg/mmol (or 30 mg/g). If albumin excretion increases even more, then it already speaks of kidney disease.

Understand your Nutritional Needs

Potassium

Potassium is a naturally occurring mineral found in nearly all foods, in varying amounts. Our bodies need an amount of potassium to help with muscle activity as well as electrolyte balance and regulation of blood pressure. However, if potassium is in excess within the system and the kidneys can't expel it (due to renal disease), fluid retention and muscle spasms can occur.

Phosphorus

Phosphorus is a trace mineral found in a wide range of foods and especially dairy, meat, and eggs. It acts synergistic ally with calcium as well as Vitamin D to promote bone health. However, when there is damage in the kidneys, excess amounts of the mineral cannot be taken out and this can cause bone weakness.

Calories

When being on a renal diet, it is vital to give yourself the right number of calories to fuel your system. The exact number of calories you should consume daily depends on your age, gender, general health status and stage of renal disease. In most cases though, there are no strict limitations in the calorie intake, as long as you take them from proper sources that are low in sodium, potassium, and phosphorus. In general, doctors recommend a daily limit between 1800-2100 calories per day to keep weight within the normal range.

Protein

Protein is an essential nutrient that our systems need to develop and generate new connective tissue e.g. muscles, even during injuries. Protein also helps stop bleeding and supports the immune system fight infections. A healthy adult with no kidney disease would usually need 40-65 grams of protein per day.

However, in renal diet, protein consumption is a tricky subject as too much or too little can cause problems. Protein, when being metabolized by our systems also creates waste which is typically processed by the kidneys. But when kidneys are damaged or underperforming, as in the case of kidney disease that waste will stay in the system. This is why patients in more advanced CKD stages are advised to limit their protein consumption as well.

Fats

Our systems need fats and particularly good fats as a fuel source and for other metabolic cell functions. A diet rich in bad and Trans or saturated fats though can significantly raise the odds of developing heart problems, which often occur with the renal disease. This is why most physicians advise their renal patients to follow a diet that contains a decent amount of good fats and a meager amount of Trans (processed) or saturated fat.

Sodium

Sodium is an essential mineral that our bodies need to regulate fluid and electrolyte balance. It also plays a role in normal cell division in the muscles and nervous system. However, in kidney disease, sodium can quickly spike at higher than normal levels and the kidneys will be unable to expel it causing fluid accumulation as a side-effect. Those who also suffer from heart problems as well should limit its consumption as it may raise blood pressure.

Carbohydrates

Carbs act as a major and quick fuel source for the body's cells. When we consume carbs, our systems turn them into glucose and then into energy for "feeding" our body cells. Carbs are generally not restricted in the renal diet. Still, some types of carbs contain dietary fiber as well, which helps regulate normal colon function and protect blood vessels from damage.

Dietary Fiber

Fiber is an important element in our system that cannot be properly digested but plays a key role in the regulation of our bowel movements and blood cell protection. The fiber in the renal diet is generally encouraged as it helps loosen up the stools, relieve constipation and bloating and protect from colon damage. However, many patients don't get enough amounts of dietary fiber per day as many of them are high in potassium or phosphorus. Fortunately, there are some good dietary fiber sources for CKD patients that have lower amounts of these minerals compared to others.

Vitamins/Minerals

Our systems, according to medical research, need at least 13 vitamins and minerals to keep our cells fully active and healthy. Patients with renal disease though are more likely to be depleted by water-soluble vitamins like B-complex and Vitamin C, as a result, or limited fluid consumption. Therefore, supplementation with these vitamins along with a renal diet program should help cover any possible vitamin deficiencies. Supplementation of fat-soluble vitamins like vitamins A, K, and E may be avoided as they can quickly build up in the system and turn toxic.

Fluids

When you are in an advanced stage of renal disease, fluid can quickly build-up and lead to problems. While it is important to keep your system well hydrated, you should avoid minerals like potassium and sodium which can trigger further fluid build-up and cause a host of other symptoms.

Foods Recommended for your Health

There are many foods that work well within the renal diet, and once you see the available variety, it will not seem as restrictive or difficult to follow. The key is focusing on the foods with a high level of nutrients, which make it easier for the kidneys to process waste by not adding too much that the body needs to discard. Balance is a major factor in maintaining and improving long-term renal function.

Garlic

An excellent, vitamin-rich food for the immune system, garlic is a tasty substitute for salt in a variety of dishes. It acts as a significant source of vitamin C and B6, while aiding the kidneys in ridding the body of unwanted toxins. It's a great, healthy way to add flavor for skillet meals, pasta, soups, and stews.

Berries

All berries are considered a good renal diet food due to their high level of fiber, antioxidants, and delicious taste, making them an easy option to include as a light snack or as an ingredient in smoothies, salads, and light desserts. Just one handful of blueberries can provide almost one day's vitamin C requirement, as well as a boost of fiber, which is good for weight loss and maintenance.

Bell Peppers

Flavorful and easy to enjoy both raw and cooked, bell peppers offer a good source of vitamin C, vitamin A, and fiber. Along with other kidney-friendly foods, they make the detoxification process much easier while boosting your body's nutrient level to prevent further health conditions and reduce existing deficiencies.

Onions

This nutritious and tasty vegetable is excellent as a companion to garlic in many dishes, or on its own. Like garlic, onions can provide flavor as an alternative to salt, and provides a good source of vitamin C, vitamin B, manganese, and fiber, as well. Adding just one quarter or half of an onion is often enough for most meals, because of its strong, pungent flavor.

Macadamia Nuts

If you enjoy nuts and seeds as snacks, you many soon learn that many contain high amounts of phosphorus and should be avoided or limited as much as possible. Fortunately, macadamia nuts are an easier option to digest and process, as they contain much lower amounts of phosphorus and make an excellent substitute for other nuts. They are a good source of other nutrients, as well, such as vitamin B, copper, manganese, iron, and healthy fats.

Pineapple

Unlike other fruits that are high in potassium, pineapple is an option that can be enjoyed more often than bananas and kiwis. Citrus fruits are generally high in potassium as well, so if you find yourself craving an orange or grapefruit, choose pineapple instead. In addition to providing a high levels of vitamin B and fiber, pineapples can reduce inflammation thanks to an enzyme called brome lain.

Mushrooms

In general, mushrooms are a safe, healthy option for the renal diet, especially the shiitake variety, which are high in nutrients such as selenium, vitamin B, and manganese. They contain a moderate amount of plant-based protein, which is easier for your body to digest and use than animal proteins. Shiitake and Portobello mushrooms are often used in vegan diets as a meat substitute, due to their texture and pleasant flavor.

Foods that are Toxic and Harmful to Health

Eating restrictions might be different depending upon your level of kidney disease. If you are in the early stages of kidney disease, you may have different restrictions as compared to those who are at the end-stage renal disease, or kidney failure. In contrast to this, people with an end-stage renal disease requiring dialysis will face different eating restrictions. Let's discuss some of the foods to avoid while being on the renal diet.

Dark-Colored Colas contain calories, sugar, phosphorus, etc. They contain phosphorus to enhance flavor, increase its life and avoid discoloration. Which can be found in a product's ingredient list. This addition of phosphorus varies depending on the type of cola. Mostly, the dark-colored colas contain 50–100 mg in a 200-ml serving. Therefore, dark colas should be avoided on a renal diet.

Canned Foods including soups, vegetables, and beans, are low in cost but contain high amounts of sodium due to the addition of salt to increase its life. Due to this amount of sodium inclusion in canned goods, it is better that people with kidney disease should avoid consumption. Opt for lower-sodium content with the label "no salt added". One more way is to drain or rinse canned foods, such as canned beans and tuna, could decrease the sodium content by 33–80%, depending on the product.

Brown Rice is a whole grain containing a higher concentration of potassium and phosphorus than its white rice counterpart. One cup already cooked brown rice possess about 150 mg of phosphorus and 154 mg of potassium, whereas, one cup of already cooked white rice has an amount of about 69 mg of phosphorus and 54 mg of potassium. Bulgur, buckwheat, pearled barley and couscous are equally beneficial, low-phosphorus options and might be a good alternative instead of brown rice.

Bananas are high potassium content, low in sodium, and provides 422 mg of potassium per banana. It might disturb your daily balanced potassium intake to 2,000 mg if a banana is a daily staple.

Whole-Wheat Bread may harm individuals with kidney disease. But for healthy individuals, it is recommended over refined, white flour bread. White bread is recommended instead of whole-wheat varieties for individuals with kidney disease just because it has phosphorus and potassium. If you add more bran and whole grains in the bread, then the amount of phosphorus and potassium contents goes higher.

Oranges and Orange Juice are enriched with vitamin C content and potassium. 184 grams provides 333 mg of potassium and 473 mg of potassium in one cup of orange juice. With these calculations, oranges and orange juice must be avoided or used in a limited amount while being on a renal diet.

Potatoes and sweet potatoes, being, the potassium-rich vegetables with 156 g contains 610 mg of potassium, whereas 114 g contains 541 mg of potassium which is relatively high. Some of the high-potassium foods, likewise potatoes and sweet potatoes, could also be soaked or leached to lessen the concentration of potassium contents. Cut them into small and thin pieces and boil those for at least 10 minutes can reduce the potassium content by about 50%. Potatoes which are soaked in a wide pot of water for as low as four hours before cooking could possess even less potassium content than those not soaked before cooking. This is known as "potassium leaching," or the "double cook Direction."

If you are suffering from or living with kidney disease, reducing your potassium, phosphorus and sodium intake is an essential aspect of managing and tackling the disease. The foods with high-potassium, high-sodium, and high-phosphorus content listed above should always be limited or avoided. These restrictions and nutrients intakes may differ depending on the level of damage to your kidneys. Following a renal diet might be a daunting procedure and a restrictive one most of the times. But, working with your physician and nutrition specialist and a renal dietitian can assist you to formulate a renal diet specific to your individual needs.

How to Manage the Renal Diet When You Are Diabetic

Patients who struggle from kidney health issues, going through kidney dialysis and have renal impairments need to not only go through medical treatment but also change their eating habit, lifestyle to make the situation better. Many researches have been done on this, and the conclusion is food has a lot to do with how your kidney functions and its overall health.

The first thing to changing your lifestyle is knowing about how your kidney functions and how different food can trigger different reactions in the kidney function. There are certain nutrients that affect your kidney directly. Nutrients like sodium, protein, phosphate, and potassium are the risky ones. You do not have to omit them altogether from your diet, but you need to limit or minimize their intake as much as possible. You cannot leave out essential nutrient like protein from your diet, but you need to count how much protein you are having per day. This is essential in order to keep balance in your muscles and maintaining a good functioning kidney.

A vast change in kidney patients is measuring how much fluid they are drinking. This is a crucial change in every kidney patient, and you must adapt to this new eating habit. Too much water or any other form of liquid can disrupt your kidney function. How much fluid you can consume depends on the condition of your kidney. Most people assign separate bottles for them so that they can measure how much they have drunk and how much more they can drink throughout the day.

Adopt a Healthy Lifestyle To Reduce The Occurrence Of Kidney Disease.

Once a kidney is damaged there is no one-time solution or magic to undo all the damage. It requires constant management and a whole new lifestyle to provide a healthy environment for your kidneys. For healthy kidneys, you just need to keep the following in mind:

Upgrade your vegetable intake to 5-9 vegetables per day.

Reduce the salt intake in your diet.

Cut down the overall protein intake.

Remove all the triggers of heart diseases, like fats and sugar, from your diet.

Do not consume pesticides and other environmental contaminants.

Try to consume fresh food; homemade is the best.

Avoid using food additives, as they contain high amounts of potassium, sodium, and phosphorous.

Drink lots of sodium-free drinks, especially water.

Choose to be more active and exercise regularly.

Do not smoke to avoid toxicity.

Obesity can create a greater risk of kidney diseases, so control your weight.

Do not take painkillers excessively, such as Ibuprofen, as they can also damage your kidneys.

Tips and Advice for Those with Kidney Disease

Tips on controlling your phosphorous

Here is what you should do to maintain a balanced level of phosphorous:

- Limit the consumption of foods like poultry, meats, fish and dairy
- Limit the intake of certain dairy products like yogurt and cheese; you should not exceed 4 oz. Per serving
- Avoid black beans, lima beans, red beans, garbanzo beans, white beans and black-eyed peas.
- Avoid unrefined, whole and dark grains.
- Stay away from refrigerator dough
- Avoid dried fruits and vegetables
- Avoid chocolate
- Avoid sodas that are dark-colored
- Make sure to take your phosphate folders with your snacks and meals.
- The renal diet limits the intake of phosphorus to 1000mg per day

Tips on Controlling your Protein

Make sure to consume high-quality proteins. Eat about 7 to 8 oz. of protein per day. Pork, beef, turkey, veal; chicken and eggs have high amounts of protein.

Tips on Controlling your Fluid Intake

- Use 1 cup or glass in order to divide your fluid intake per day. You can also write a record of your fluid intake.
- Always avoid any type of salty food and never add extra salt to your meals.
- Avoid processed meats, fast foods and canned foods
- You can add lemon juice to the water you want to drink instead
- You can clean your mouth with a mouthwash from time to time
- Avoid overheating
- Maintain your blood sugar at a balanced level

Eating Out

Look out for small or half portions and ask your server for your foods to be cooked without extra salt, butter or sauce. Avoid fried foods, instead, embrace poached or grilled food. If you know, you are going out to eat, plan ahead. Look at the restaurant menu beforehand online.

Eating at social gatherings (such as birthdays, weddings, picnics, and barbecues)

1. Don't go hungry: Have a snack before you leave the house.

2. Avoid high-sodium foods: Avoid foods such as hot dogs or sausages. Choose lower-sodium foods such as chicken and hamburgers.

3. Limit alcohol: Speak with your physician first about drinking alcohol.

4. Plan ahead: Plan your menus.

Meat

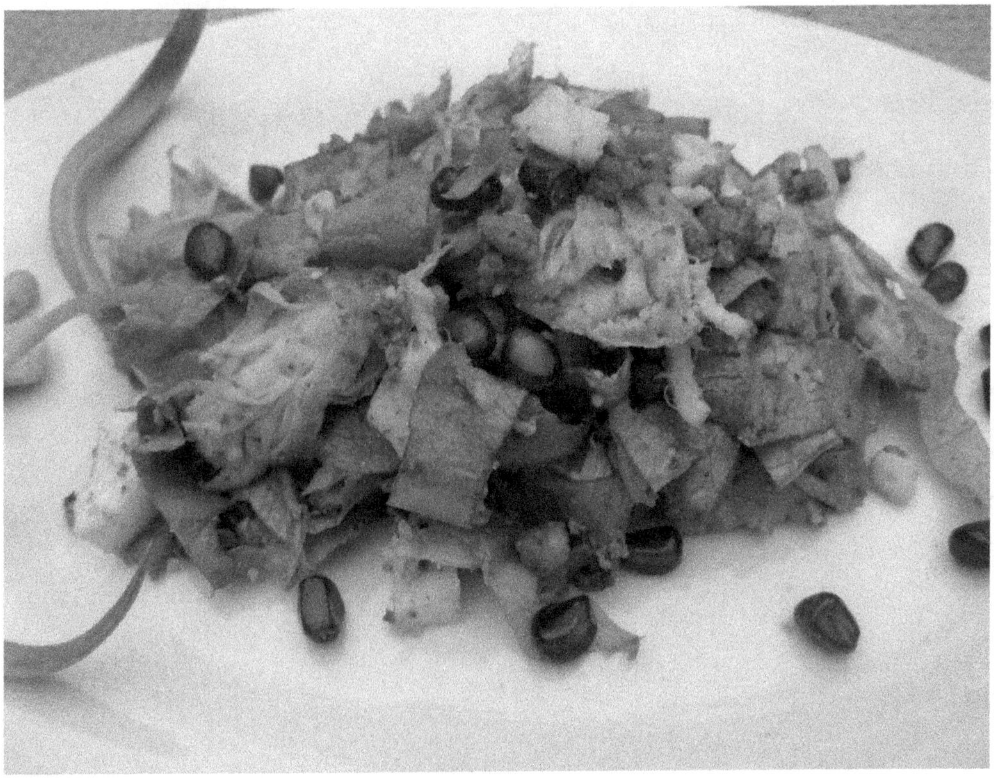

Peppercorn Pork Chops

Preparation time: 20 minutes
Cooking Time: 25 minutes
Servings: 4

Ingredients:

- 1 tablespoon crushed black peppercorns
- 4 pork loin chops
- 2 tablespoons olive oil
- 1/4 cup butter
- 5 garlic cloves
- 1 cup green and red bell peppers
- 1/2 cup pineapple juice

Directions:

1. Sprinkle and press peppercorns into both sides of pork chops.
2. Heat oil, butter and garlic cloves in a large skillet over medium heat, stirring frequently.
3. Add pork chops and cook uncovered for 5-6 minutes.
4. Dice the bell peppers. Add the bell peppers and pineapple juice to the pork chops.
5. Cover and simmer for another 5-6 minutes or until pork is thoroughly cooked.

Nutrition:

Calories 317,

Sodium 126mg,

Dietary Fiber 2g,

Total Sugars 6.4g,

Protein 13.2g,

Calcium 39mg,

Potassium 250mg,

Phosphorus 115 mg

Pork Chops with Apples, Onions

Preparation time: 25 minutes
Cooking Time: 55 minutes
Servings: 4

Ingredients:

- 4 pork chops
- salt and pepper to taste
- 2 onions, sliced into rings
- 2 apples - peeled, cored, and sliced into rings
- 3 tablespoons honey
- 2 teaspoons freshly ground black pepper

Directions:

1. Preheat oven to 375 degrees F.

2. Spice pork chops with salt and pepper to taste, and arrange in a medium oven-safe skillet. Top pork chops with onions and apples. Sprinkle with honey. Season with 2 teaspoons pepper.

3. Cover, and bake 1 hour in the preheated oven, pork chops have reached an internal temperature of 145 degrees F.

Nutrition:

Calories 307,

Sodium 48mg,

Dietary Fiber 3.1g,

Total Sugars 21.5g,

Protein 15.1g,

Calcium 30mg,

Potassium 387mg,

Phosphorus 315 mg

Beef Patties

Preparation Time: 10 minutes

Cooking Time: 8 minutes

Servings: 5

Ingredients:

- 1 lb ground beef
- 1 egg, lightly beaten
- 3 tablespoon almond flour
- 1 small onion, grated
- 2 tablespoon fresh parsley, chopped
- 1 teaspoon dry oregano
- 1 teaspoon dry mint
- Pepper
- Salt

Directions:

1. Mix all ingredients in a container till combined.
2. Make small patties from the meat mixture.
3. Heat grill pan over medium-high heat.
4. Place patties in a hot pan and cook for 4-5 minutes on each side.
5. Serve and enjoy.

Nutrition:

Calories 188

Fat 6.6 g

Carbohydrates 1.7 g

Sugar 0.7 g

Protein 28.9 g

Cholesterol 114 mg

Calcium 79mg,

Phosphorous 316mg,

Potassium 227mg

Sodium: 121 mg

Roasted Sirloin Steak

Preparation Time: 10 minutes
Cooking Time: 30 minutes
Servings: 6
Ingredients:

- 2 lbs sirloin steak, cut into 1" cubes
- 2 garlic cloves, minced
- 3 tablespoon fresh lemon juice
- 1 teaspoon dried oregano
- 1/4 cup water
- 1/4 cup olive oil
- 2 cups fresh parsley, chopped
- 1/2 teaspoon pepper
- 1 teaspoon salt

Directions:

1. Add all ingredients except beef into the large bowl and mix well.
2. Pour bowl mixture into the large zip-lock bag.
3. Add beef to the bag and jiggle well and refrigerate for 1 hour.
4. Preheat the oven 400 F.
5. Place marinated beef on a baking tray and bake in preheated oven for 30 minutes.
6. Serve and enjoy.

Nutrition:
Calories 365
Fat 18.1 g
Carbohydrates 2 g
Sugar 0.4 g
Protein 46.6 g
Cholesterol 135 mg
Calcium 79mg,
Phosphorous 266mg,
Potassium 204mg
Sodium: 178 mg

Meatballs

Preparation Time: 10 minutes
Cooking Time: 4 hours
Servings: 6
Ingredients:

- 1 egg
- 2 tablespoon fresh parsley, chopped
- 1 garlic clove, minced
- ½ lb ground beef
- ½ lb ground pork
- 14 oz can tomatoes, crushed
- 2 tablespoon fresh basil, chopped
- ¼ teaspoon pepper
- ½ teaspoon salt

Directions:

1. In a mixing bowl, mix together beef, pork, egg, parsley, garlic, pepper, and salt until well combined.
2. Make small balls from meat mixture.
3. Arrange meatballs into the slow cooker.
4. Pour crushed tomatoes, basil, pepper, and salt over meatballs.
5. Cover and cook on low for 4 hours.
6. Serve and enjoy.

Nutrition:

Calories 150
Fat 4 g
Carbohydrates 4 g
Sugar 2 g
Protein 24 g
Cholesterol 90 mg
Calcium 67mg,
Phosphorous 76mg,
Potassium 88mg
Sodium: 134 mg

Shredded Beef

Preparation time: 10 minutes
Cooking Time: 5 hr.10 minutes
Servings: 4
Ingredients:

- 1/2 cup onion
- 2 garlic cloves
- 2 tablespoons fresh parsley
- 2-pound beef rump roast
- 1 tablespoon Italian herb seasoning
- 1 teaspoon dried parsley
- 1 bay leaf
- 1/2 teaspoon pepper
- 1/4 teaspoon salt
- 2 tablespoons olive oil
- 1/3 cup vinegar
- 2 to 3 cups water
- 8 hard rolls, 3-1/2-inch diameter, 2 ounces each

Directions:

1. Chop onion, garlic and fresh parsley. Place beef roast in a Crock-Pot. Add chopped onion, garlic and remaining ingredients, except fresh parsley and rolls, to Crock-Pot; stir to combine.
2. Over low-heat setting, cover and cook for 8 to 10 hours, or on high setting for 4 to 5 hours, until fork-tender.
3. Remove roast from Crock-Pot.
4. Shred with two forks then return meat to cooking broth to keep warm until ready to serve.
5. Slice rolls in half and top with shredded beef, fresh parsley and 1-2 spoons of the broth.
6. Serve open-face or as a sandwich.

Nutrition:
Calories 218,
Sodium 184mg,
Dietary Fiber 0.4g,
Total Sugars 0.4g,
Protein 26g,
Calcium 26mg,
Potassium 28mg,
Phosphorus 30mg

Lamb Stew with Green Beans

Preparation time: 30 minutes
Cooking Time: 1 hr.10 minutes
Servings: 4
Ingredients:

- 1 tablespoon olive oil
- 1 large onion, chopped
- 1 stalk green onion, chopped
- 1-pound boneless lamb shoulder, cut into 2-inch pieces
- 3 cups hot water
- ½ pound fresh green beans, trimmed
- 1 tablespoon chopped fresh parsley
- 1/2 teaspoon dried mint
- 1/2 teaspoon dried dill weed
- 1 pinch ground nutmeg
- ¼ teaspoon honey
- Salt and pepper to taste

Directions:

1. In a large pot over moderate temperature, heat oil. Sauté onion and green onion until golden.
2. Stir in lamb, and cook until evenly brown.
3. Stir in water. Reduce heat and simmer for about 1 hour.
4. Stir in green beans. Season with parsley, mint, dill, nutmeg, honey, salt and pepper.
5. Continue cooking until beans are tender.

Nutrition:
Calories 81,
Sodium 20mg,
Dietary Fiber 1g,
Total Sugars 1g,
Protein 6.5g,
Calcium 17mg,
Potassium 136mg,
Phosphorus 120mg

Laurel Lamb with Oregano

Preparation Time: 5 minutes

Cooking Time: 30 minutes

Servings: 4

Ingredients:

- 1,65 lb lamb chops
- 3 cloves garlic
- 3 leaves laurel
- A sprig of oregano
- 2 tablespoons chopped parsley
- 1 tablespoon fresh or dried rosemary
- C / N virgin olive oil

Directions:

1. Put the chops on a platter and sprinkle with herbs and garlic, peeled and chopped. Add salt and pepper and marinate overnight.
2. The next day put the meat in a bowl and sprinkle with olive aciete. Leave to marinate at least 4 hours. Place all in a baking dish and close either with transparent foil.
3. Preheat air fryer to 282 ° F for 1
4. Lowering the temperature to 338 ° F and leave about 15'.
5. Now remove meat from the Air fryer and raise the temperature of Air fryer to 428 ° F.
6. Remove the plastic wrap and return to the Air fryer for a few minutes until the meat has a golden color.
7. Serve with roasted or fried potatoes.

Nutrition:

Calories: 206

Fat: 21.3g

Carbs: 15g

Protein: 13g

Calcium 79mg,

Phosphorous 216mg,

Potassium 127mg

Sodium: 121 mg

Lamb Keema

Preparation time: 10 minutes
Cooking Time: 15 minutes
Servings: 4
Ingredients:

- 1 1/2 pounds ground lamb
- 1 onion, finely chopped
- 2 teaspoons garlic powder
- 2 tablespoons garam masala
- 1/8 teaspoon salt
- 3/4 cup chicken broth

Directions:

1. In a large, heavy skillet over average heat, cook ground lamb until evenly brown.
2. While cooking, break apart with a wooden spoon until crumbled.
3. Transfer cooked lamb to a bowl and drain off all but 1 tablespoon fat. Sauté onion until soft and translucent, about 5 minutes.
4. Stir in garlic powder, and sauté 1 minute.
5. Stir in garam masala and cook 1 minute.
6. Return the browned lamb to the pan, and stir in chicken beef broth.
7. Reduce heat, and simmer for 10 to 15 minutes or until meat is fully cooked through, and liquid has evaporated.

Nutrition:
Calories 194,
Sodium 160mg,
Total Carbohydrate 2.2g,
Dietary Fiber 0.4g,
Total Sugars 0.9g,
Protein 28.1g,
Calcium 18mg,
Potassium 379mg,
Phosphorus 240mg

Beef with Beans

Preparation Time: 10 Minutes

Cooking Time: 13 Minutes

Servings: 4

Ingredients:

- 12 Oz. Lean Steak
- 1 Onion, sliced
- 1 Can Chopped Tomatoes
- 3/4 Cup Beef Stock
- 4 Tsp Fresh Thyme, chopped
- 1 Can Red Kidney Beans
- Salt and Pepper to taste
- Oven Safe Bowl

Directions:

1. Preheat the Cuisinart Air Fryer Oven to 390 degrees.
2. Fryer Oven. Set temperature to 390°F, and set time to 13 minutes, Cook for 3 minutes. Add the meat and continue cooking for 5 minutes.
3. Add the tomatoes and their juice, beef stock, thyme and the beans and cook for an additional 5 minutes
4. Season with black pepper to taste.

Nutrition:

Calories: 178

Fat: 14g

Protein: 9g

Fiber: 0g

Calcium 29mg,

Phosphorous 116mg,

Potassium 202mg

Sodium: 131 mg

Easy Pork Kabobs

Preparation Time: 10 minutes
Cooking Time: 4 hours 20 minutes
Servings: 6
Ingredients:

- 2 lbs pork tenderloin, cut into 1-inch cubes
- 1 onion, chopped
- ½ cup olive oil
- ½ cup red wine vinegar
- 2 tablespoon fresh parsley, chopped
- 2 garlic cloves, chopped
- Pepper
- Salt

Directions:

1. In a large zip-lock bag, mix together red wine vinegar, parsley, garlic, onion, and oil.
2. Add meat to bag and marinate in the refrigerator for overnight.
3. Remove marinated pork from refrigerator and thread onto soaked wooden skewers. Season with pepper and salt.
4. Preheat the grill over high heat.
5. Grill pork for 3-4 minutes on both side.
6. Serve and enjoy.

Nutrition:
Calories 375
Fat 22 g
Carbohydrates 2.5 g
Sugar 1 g
Protein 40 g
Cholesterol 110 mg
Calcium 34mg,
Phosphorous 136mg,
Potassium 127mg
Sodium: 121 mg

Lamb Barley Soup

Preparation time: 20 minutes

Cooking Time: 60 minutes

Servings: 4

Ingredients:

- 1-pound ground lamb
- 1/2 large onion, chopped
- 2 cups water
- 4 medium carrots, chopped
- 3 stalks celery, chopped
- 1/2 cup barley
- 1/2 teaspoon chili powder
- 1/2 teaspoon ground black pepper

Directions:

1. Heat a big skillet over medium-high warmth and stir in the ground lamb and onion.
2. Cook and stir until the lamb is evenly browned and onions are translucent.
3. Drain and discard any excess grease.
4. Add water, the carrots, celery, and barley, and season with chili powder and pepper.
5. Simmer over medium heat for 45 minutes.

Nutrition:

Calories 79,

Sodium 39mg,

Total Carbohydrate 12.7g,

Dietary Fiber 3.1g,

Total Sugars 2.1g,

Protein 4.8g,

Calcium 23mg,

Iron 1mg,

Potassium 221mg,

Phosphorus 170mg

Feta Lamb Patties

Preparation Time: 10 minutes

Cooking Time: 12 minutes

Servings: 4

Ingredients:

- 1 lb ground lamb
- 1/2 teaspoon garlic powder
- 1/2 cup feta cheese, crumbled
- 1/4 cup mint leaves, chopped
- 1/4 cup roasted red pepper, chopped
- 1/4 cup onion, chopped
- Pepper
- Salt

Directions:

1. Add all ingredients into the container and mix until well combined.
2. Spray pan with cooking spray and heat over medium-high heat.
3. Make small patties from meat mixture and place on hot pan and cook for 6-7 minutes on each side.
4. Serve and enjoy.

Nutrition:

Calories 270

Fat 12 g

Carbohydrates 2.9 g

Sugar 1.7 g

Protein 34.9 g

Cholesterol 119 mg

Calcium 49mg,

Phosphorous 116mg,

Potassium 137mg

Sodium: 121 mg

Simple Steak

Preparation Time: 6minutes

Cooking Time: 14 Minutes

Servings: 2

Ingredients:

- ½ pound quality cuts steak
- Salt and freshly ground black pepper, to taste

Directions:

1. Preheat the air fryer to 390 degrees F.
2. Rub the steak with salt and pepper evenly.
3. Place the steak in the air fryer basket and cook for about 14 minutes crispy.

Nutrition:

Calories: 198

Fat: 7g

Protein: 43g

Fiber: 0g

Calcium 79mg,

Phosphorous 126mg,

Potassium 107mg

Sodium: 131 mg

Creamy Turkey

Preparation time: 12 minutes
Cooking Time: 10 minutes
Servings: 4

Ingredients:

- 4 skinless, boneless turkey breast halves
- Salt and pepper to taste
- ½ teaspoon ground black pepper
- ½ teaspoon garlic powder
- 1 (10.75 ounces) can chicken soup

Directions:

1. Preheat oven to 375 degrees F.

2. Clean turkey breasts and season with salt, pepper and garlic powder (or whichever seasonings you prefer) on both sides of turkey pieces.

3. Bake for 25 minutes, then add chicken soup and bake for 10 more minutes (or until done). Serve over rice or egg noodles.

Nutrition:

Calories 160,

Sodium 157mg,

Dietary Fiber 0.4g,

Total Sugars 0.4g,

Protein 25.6g,

Calcium 2mg,

Potassium 152mg,

Phosphorus 85 mg

Lemon Pepper Chicken Legs

Preparation Time: 5 minutes

Cooking Time: 25 minutes

Servings: 4

Ingredients:

- ½ tsp. garlic powder
- 2 tsp. baking powder
- 8 chicken legs
- 4 tbsp. salted butter, melted
- 1 tbsp. lemon pepper seasoning

Directions:

1. In a small container add the garlic powder and baking powder, then use this mixture to coat the chicken legs. Lay the chicken in the basket of your fryer.
2. Cook the chicken legs at 375°F for twenty-five minutes. Halfway through, turn them over and allow to cook on the other side.
3. When the chicken has turned golden brown, test with a thermometer to ensure it has reached an ideal temperature of 165°F. Remove from the fryer.
4. Mix together the melted butter and lemon pepper seasoning and toss with the chicken legs until the chicken is coated all over. Serve hot.

Nutrition:

Calories: 132

Fat: 16 g

Carbs: 20 g

Protein: 48 g

Calcium 79mg,

Phosphorous 132mg,

Potassium 127mg

Sodium: 121 mg

Turkey Broccoli Salad

Preparation time: 10 minutes
Cooking Time: 00 minutes
Servings: 4

Ingredients:

- 8 cups broccoli florets
- 3 cooked skinless, boneless chicken breast halves, cubed
- 6 green onions, chopped
- 1 cup mayonnaise
- ¼ cup apple cider vinegar
- ¼ cup honey

Directions:

1. Combine broccoli, chicken and green onions in a large bowl.
2. Whisk mayonnaise, vinegar, and honey together in a bowl until well blended.
3. Pour mayonnaise dressing over broccoli mixture; toss to coat.
4. Cover and refrigerate until chilled, if desired. Serve

Nutrition:

Calories 133,

Sodium 23mg,

Dietary Fiber 1.6g,

Total Sugars 7.7g,

Protein 6.2g,

Calcium 24mg,

Potassium 157mg

Phosphorus 148 mg

Fruity Chicken Salad

Preparation time: 10 minutes
Cooking Time: 5 minutes
Servings: 3

Ingredients:

- 4 skinless, boneless chicken breast halves - cooked and diced
- 1 stalk celery, diced
- 4 green onions, chopped
- 1 Golden Delicious apple - peeled, cored and diced
- 1/3 cup seedless green grapes, halved
- 1/8 teaspoon ground black pepper
- 3/4 cup light mayonnaise

Directions:

1. In a large container, add the celery, chicken, onion, apple, grapes, pepper, and mayonnaise.

2. Mix all together. Serve!

Nutrition:

Calories 196,

Sodium 181mg,

Total Carbohydrate 15.6g,

Dietary Fiber 1.2g,

Total Sugars 9.1g,

Protein 13.2g,

Calcium 13mg,

Iron 1mg,

Potassium 115mg,

Phosphorus 88 mg

Buckwheat Salad

Preparation time: 12 minutes
Cooking Time: 20 minutes
Servings: 3
Ingredients:

- 2 cups water
- 1 clove garlic, smashed
- 1 cup uncooked buckwheat
- 2 large cooked chicken breasts - cut into bite-size pieces
- 1 large red onion, diced
- 1 large green bell pepper, diced
- 1/4 cup chopped fresh parsley
- 1/4 cup chopped fresh chives
- 1/2 teaspoon salt
- 2/3 cup fresh lemon juice
- 1 tablespoon balsamic vinegar
- 1/4 cup olive oil

Directions:

1. Bring the water, garlic to a boil in a saucepan. Stir in the buckwheat, reduce heat to medium-low, cover, and simmer until the buckwheat is tender and the water has been absorbed, 15 to 20 minutes.
2. Discard the garlic clove and scrape the buckwheat into a large bowl.
3. Gently stir the chicken, onion, bell pepper, parsley, chives, and salt into the buckwheat.
4. Sprinkle with the olive oil, balsamic vinegar, and lemon juice. Stir until evenly mixed.

Nutrition:
Calories 199,
Total Fat 8.3g,
Sodium 108mg,
Dietary Fiber 2.9g,
Total Sugars 2g,
Protein 13.6g,
Calcium 22mg,
Potassium 262mg,
Phosphorus 188 mg

Vegetables

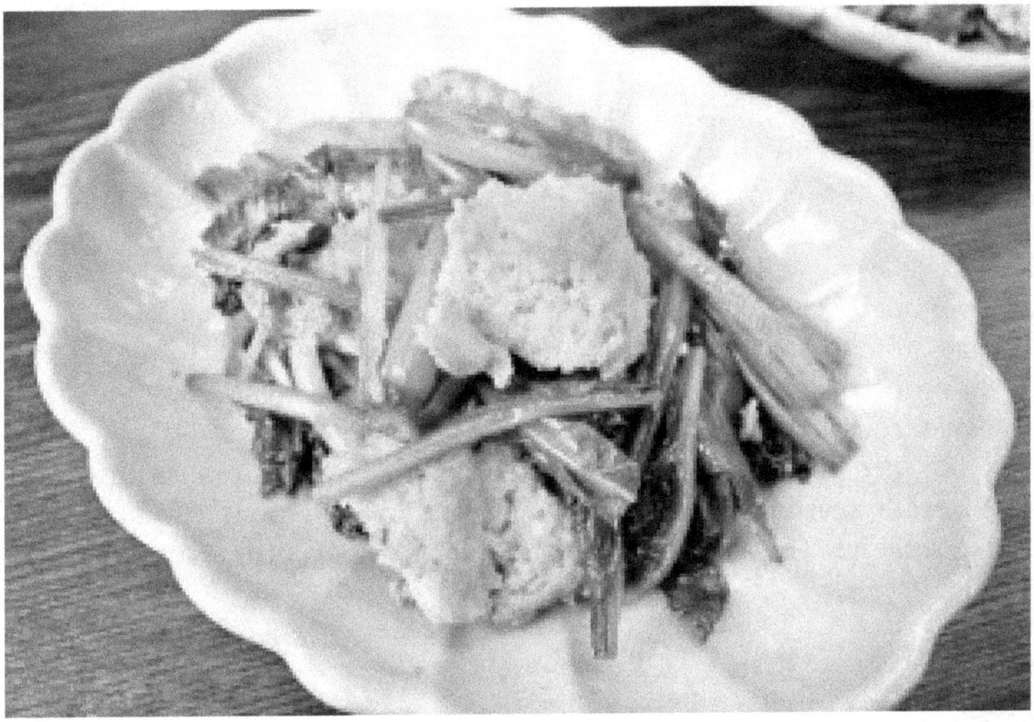

Curried Veggie Stir-Fry

Preparation Time: 20 minutes
Cooking Time: 10 minutes
Servings: 6
Ingredients:

- 2 tablespoons of extra-virgin olive oil
- 1 onion, chopped
- 4 garlic cloves, minced
- 4 cups of frozen stir-fry vegetables
- 1 cup of canned unsweetened full-fat coconut milk
- 1 cup of water
- 2 tablespoons of green curry paste

Directions:

1. In a wok or non-stick, heat the olive oil over medium-high heat. Stir-fry the onion and garlic for 2 to 3 minutes, until fragrant.
2. Add the frozen stir-fry vegetables and continue to cook for 3 to 4 minutes longer, or until the vegetables are hot.
3. Meanwhile, in a small bowl, combine coconut milk, water, and curry paste. Stir until the paste dissolves.
4. Add the broth mixture to the wok and cook for another 2 to 3 minutes, or until the sauce has reduced slightly and all the vegetables are crisp-tender.
5. Serve over couscous or hot cooked rice.

Ingredient Tip: When you buy frozen stir-fry vegetables, make sure you purchase a variety that doesn't include seasonings or sauce, which would increase the sodium content. You could also use separate veggies; try a combination of broccoli with carrots or asparagus with zucchini.

Nutrition:
Calories: 293
Total fat: 18g
Saturated fat: 10g
Sodium: 247mg
Phosphorus: 138mg
Potassium: 531mg
Carbohydrates: 28g
Fiber: 7g
Protein: 7g
Sugar: 4g

Chilaquiles

Preparation Time: 20 minutes
Cooking Time: 20 minutes
Servings: 4
Ingredients:

- 3 (8-inch) corn tortillas, cut into strips
- 2 tablespoons of extra-virgin olive oil
- 12 tomatillos, papery covering removed, chopped
- 3 tablespoons of freshly squeezed lime juice
- 1/8 teaspoon of salt
- 1/8 teaspoon of freshly ground black pepper
- 4 large egg whites
- 2 large eggs
- 2 tablespoons of water
- 1 cup of shredded pepper jack cheese

Directions:

1. In a dry nonstick skillet, toast the tortilla strips over medium heat until they are crisp, tossing the pan and stirring occasionally. This should take 4 to 6 minutes. Remove the strips from the pan and set aside.
2. In the same skillet, heat the olive oil over medium heat and add the tomatillos, lime juice, salt, and pepper. Cook and frequently stir for about 8 to 10 minutes until the tomatillos start to break down and form a sauce. Transfer the sauce to a bowl and set aside.
3. In a small bowl, beat the egg whites, eggs, and water and add to the skillet. Cook the eggs for 3 to 4 minutes, stirring occasionally until they are set and cooked to 160°F.
4. Preheat the oven to 400°F.
5. Toss the tortilla strips in the tomatillo sauce and place in a casserole dish. Top with the scrambled eggs and cheese.
6. Bake for 10 to 15 minutes, or until the cheese starts to brown. Serve.

Nutrition:
Calories: 312
Total fat: 20g
Saturated fat: 8g
Sodium: 345mg
Phosphorus: 280mg
Potassium: 453mg
Carbohydrates: 19g
Fiber: 3g
Protein: 15g
Sugar: 5g

Roasted Veggie Sandwiches

Preparation Time: 20 minutes
Cooking Time: 35 minutes
Servings: 6
Ingredients:

- 3 bell peppers, assorted colors, sliced
- 1 cup of sliced yellow summer squash
- 1 red onion, sliced
- 2 tablespoons of extra-virgin olive oil
- 2 tablespoons of balsamic vinegar
- 1/8 teaspoon of salt
- 1/8 teaspoon of freshly ground black pepper
- 3 large whole-wheat pita breads, halved

Directions:

1. Preheat the oven to 400°F.
2. Prepare a parchment paper and line it in a rimmed baking sheet.
3. Spread the bell peppers, squash, and onion on the prepared baking sheet. Sprinkle with the olive oil, vinegar, salt, and pepper.
4. Roast for 30 to 40 minutes, turning the vegetables with a spatula once during cooking, until they are tender and light golden brown.
5. Pile the vegetables into the pita breads and serve.

Ingredient Tip: Pita breads are puffed rounds that have a natural pocket in the center that holds a filling. To prepare them, cut in half crosswise and gently separate the two halves, cutting the pocket if necessary. You can find pita breads in most supermarkets.
Nutrition:
Calories: 182
Total fat: 5g
Saturated fat: 1g
Sodium: 234mg
Phosphorus: 106mg
Potassium: 289mg
Carbohydrates: 31g
Fiber: 4g
Protein: 5g
Sugar: 6g

Roasted Peach Open-Face Sandwich

Preparation Time: 5 minutes
Cooking Time: 15 minutes
Servings: 4
Ingredients:

- 2 fresh peaches, peeled and sliced
- 1 tablespoon of extra-virgin olive oil
- 1 tablespoon of freshly squeezed lemon juice
- 1/8 teaspoon of salt
- 1/8 teaspoon of freshly ground black pepper
- 4 ounces of cream cheese, at room temperature
- 2 teaspoons of fresh thyme leaves
- 4 whole-wheat sourdough bread slices

Directions:

1. Preheat the oven to 400°F.
2. Arrange the peaches on a rimmed baking sheet. Brush them with olive oil on both sides.
3. Roast the peaches for 10 to 15 minutes, until they are lightly golden brown around the edges. Sprinkle with lemon juice, salt, and pepper.
4. In a small bowl, combine the cream cheese and thyme and mix well.
5. Toast the bread. Get the toasted bread and spread it with the cream cheese mixture. Top with the peaches and serve.

Nutrition:
Calories: 250
Total fat: 13g
Saturated fat: 6g
Sodium: 376mg
Phosphorus: 163mg
Potassium: 260mg
Carbohydrates: 28g
Fiber: 3g
Protein: 6g
Sugar: 8g

Pasta Fagioli

Preparation Time: 25 minutes
Cooking Time: 25 minutes
Servings: 6
Ingredients:

- 1 (15-ounce) can low-sodium great northern beans, drained and rinsed, divided
- 2 cups frozen peppers and onions, thawed, divided
- 5 cups low-sodium vegetable broth
- 1/8 teaspoon salt
- 1/8 teaspoon freshly ground black pepper
- 1 cup whole-grain orecchiette pasta
- 2 tablespoons extra-virgin olive oil
- 1/3cup grated Parmesan cheese

Directions:

1. In a large saucepan, place the beans and cover with water. Bring to a boil over high heat and boil for 10 minutes. Drain the beans.
2. In a food processor or blender, combine 1/3cup of beans and 1/3cup of thawed peppers and onions. Process until smooth.
3. In the same saucepan, combine the pureed mixture, the remaining 1 2/3 cups of peppers and onions, the remaining beans, the broth, and the salt and pepper and bring to a simmer.
4. Add the pasta to the saucepan. Make sure to stir it and bring it to boil, reduce the heat to low, and simmer for 8 to 10 minutes, or until the pasta is tender.
5. Serve drizzled with olive oil and topped with Parmesan cheese.

Nutrition:
Calories: 245
Total fat: 7g
Saturated fat: 2g
Sodium: 269mg
Phosphorus: 188mg
Potassium: 592mg
Carbohydrates: 36g
Fiber: 7g
Protein: 12g
Sugar: 4g

Spinach Alfredo Lasagna Rolls

Preparation Time: 25 minutes
Cooking Time: 50 minutes
Servings: 4
Ingredients:

- 4 whole-grain lasagna noodles
- 2 tablespoons of extra-virgin olive oil
- 1 large onion, chopped
- 2 cups of frozen whole-leaf spinach, thawed (measure while frozen)
- 1 (8-ounce) cream cheese, divided
- 1/3cup of shredded Parmesan cheese

Directions:

1. Bring a large pot of water to a boil over high heat and add the lasagna noodles. Simmer for 8 to 9 minutes or until the pasta is almost al dente but still has a thin white line in the center. Drain, reserving ¼ cup of the pasta water, and set aside.
2. Meanwhile, in a saucepan, heat the olive oil over medium heat. Add the onions and cook for 6 to 8 minutes, stirring, until the onions are tender and starting to turn brown.
3. While the onions are cooking, drain the spinach and put the leaves into some paper towels. Squeeze well to remove most of the water from the spinach.
4. Add the spinach to the onions, stir, and turn off the heat. Add 6 ounces of cream cheese to the vegetables and stir until combined. Set aside.
5. In a small saucepan, combine the remaining 2 ounces of cream cheese with the reserved pasta water. Heat over low heat, often stirring with a wire whisk, until smooth.
6. In a 9-inch baking sheet, place 2 tablespoons of the cream cheese sauce.
7. On a work surface, place the lasagna noodles. Divide the spinach mixture among them and roll them up.
8. Place the rolls, seam-side down, on the sauce in the casserole. Top with the remaining sauce.
9. Sprinkle the lasagna rolls with the Parmesan cheese. Bake for 25 to 35 minutes, or until the lasagna is bubbling and the top starts to brown.

Nutrition:
Calories: 388
Total fat: 24g
Saturated fat: 7g
Sodium: 411mg
Phosphorus: 119mg
Potassium: 378mg
Carbohydrates: 34g
Fiber: 9g
Protein: 13g
Sugar: 5g

Spicy Corn and Rice Burritos

Preparation Time: 10 minutes
Cooking Time: 20 minutes
Servings: 4
Ingredients:

- 3 tablespoons of extra-virgin olive oil, divided
- 1 (10-ounce) package of frozen cooked brown rice
- 1½ cups of frozen yellow corn
- 1 tablespoon of chili powder
- 1 cup of shredded pepper jack cheese
- 4 large or 6 small corn tortillas

Directions:

1. Put the skillet in over medium heat and put 2 tablespoons of olive oil. Add the rice, corn, and chili powder and cook for 4 to 6 minutes, or until the ingredients are hot.
2. Transfer the ingredients from the pan into a medium bowl. Let cool for 15 minutes.
3. Stir the cheese into the rice mixture.
4. Heat the tortillas using the directions from the package to make them pliable. Fill the corn tortillas with the rice mixture, then roll them up.
5. At this point, you can serve them as is, or you can fry them first. Heat the remaining tablespoon of olive oil in a large skillet. Fry the burritos, seam-side down at first, turning once, until they are brown and crisp, about 4 to 6 minutes per side, then serve.

Nutrition:
Calories: 386
Total fat: 21g
Saturated fat: 7g
Sodium: 510mg
Phosphorus: 304mg
Potassium: 282mg
Carbohydrates: 41g
Fiber: 4g
Protein: 11g
Sugar: 2g

Crust less Cabbage Quiche

Preparation Time: 10 minutes
Cooking Time: 40 minutes
Servings: 6
Ingredients:

- Olive oil cooking spray
- 2 tablespoons of extra-virgin olive oil
- 3 cups of coleslaw blend with carrots
- 3 large eggs, beaten
- 3 large egg whites, beaten
- ½ cup of half-and-half
- 1 teaspoon of dried dill weed
- 1/8 teaspoon of salt
- 1/8 teaspoon of freshly ground black pepper
- 1 cup of grated Swiss cheese

Directions:

1. Preheat the oven to 350°F. Spray pie plate (9-inch) with cooking spray and set aside.
2. In a skillet, put an oil and put it in medium heat. Add the coleslaw mix and cook for 4 to 6 minutes, stirring, until the cabbage is tender. Transfer the vegetables from the pan to a medium bowl to cool.
3. Meanwhile, in another medium bowl, combine the eggs and egg whites, half-and-half, dill, salt, and pepper and beat to combine.
4. Stir the cabbage mixture into the egg mixture and pour into the prepared pie plate.
5. Sprinkle with the cheese.
6. Bake for 30 to 35 minutes, or until the mixture is puffed, set, and light golden brown. Let stand for 5 minutes, then slice to serve.

Nutrition:
Calories: 203
Total fat: 16g
Saturated fat: 6g
Sodium: 321mg
Phosphorus: 169mg
Potassium: 155mg
Carbohydrates: 5g
Fiber: 1g
Protein: 11g
Sugar: 4g

Creamy Veggie Casserole

Preparation Time: 25 minutes
Cooking Time: 35 minutes
Servings: 4
Ingredients:

- 1/3cup of extra-virgin olive oil, divided
- 1 onion, chopped
- 2 tablespoons of flour
- 3 cups of low-sodium vegetable broth
- 3 cups of frozen California blend vegetables
- 1 cup of crushed crisp rice cereal

Directions:

1. Preheat the oven to 375°F.
2. Next is heat 2 tablespoons of olive oil in a large skillet over medium heat. Add the onion and cook for 3 to 4 minutes, stirring, until the onion is tender.
3. Add the flour and stir for 2 minutes.
4. Add the broth to the saucepan, stirring for 3 to 4 minutes, or until the sauce starts to thicken.
5. Add the vegetables to the saucepan. Simmer and cook until vegetables are tender (for six to eight minutes).
6. When the vegetables are done, pour the mixture into a 3-quart casserole dish.
7. Sprinkle the vegetables with the crushed cereal.
8. Bake for 20 to 25 minutes or until the cereal is golden brown and the filling is bubbling. Let cool for 5 minutes and serve.

Nutrition:
Calories: 234
Total fat: 18g
Saturated fat: 3g
Sodium: 139mg
Phosphorus: 21mg
Potassium: 210mg
Carbohydrates: 16g
Fiber: 3g
Protein: 3g
Sugar: 5g

Vegetable Green Curry

Preparation Time: 20 minutes

Cooking Time: 20 minutes

Servings: 6

Ingredients:

- 2 tablespoons of extra-virgin olive oil
- 1 head of broccoli, cut into florets
- 1 bunch of asparagus, cut into 2-inch lengths
- 3 tablespoons of water
- 2 tablespoons of green curry paste
- 1 medium eggplant
- 1/8 teaspoon of salt
- 1/8 teaspoon of freshly ground black pepper
- 2/3 cup of plain whole-milk yogurt

Directions:

1. Put olive oil in a large saucepan in medium heat. Add the broccoli and stir-fry for 5 minutes. Add the asparagus and stir-fry for another 3 minutes.
2. Meanwhile, in a small bowl, combine the water with the green curry paste.
3. Add the eggplant, curry-water mixture, salt, and pepper. Stir-fry or until vegetables are all tender.
4. Add the yogurt. Heat through but avoid simmering. Serve.

Nutrition:

Calories: 113

Total fat: 6g

Saturated fat: 1g

Sodium: 174mg

Phosphorus: 117mg

Potassium: 569mg

Carbohydrates: 13g

Fiber: 6g

Protein: 5g

Sugar: 7g

Zucchini Bowl

Preparation Time: 10 minutes

Cooking Time: 20 minutes

Servings: 4

Ingredients:

- 1 onion, chopped
- 3 zucchini, cut into medium chunks
- 2 tablespoons coconut milk
- 2 garlic cloves, minced
- 4 cups chicken stock
- 2 tablespoons coconut oil
- Pinch of salt
- Black pepper to taste

Directions:

1. Take a pot and place it over medium heat
2. Add oil and let it heat up
3. Add zucchini, garlic, onion, and stir
4. Cook for 5 minutes
5. Add stock, salt, pepper, and stir
6. Bring to a boil and lower down the heat
7. Simmer for 20 minutes.
8. Remove heat and add coconut milk
9. Use an immersion blender until smooth
10. Ladle into soup bowls and serve
11. Enjoy!

Nutrition:

Calories: 160

Fat: 2g

Carbohydrates: 4g

Protein: 7g

Nice Coconut Haddock

Preparation Time: 10 minutes

Cooking Time: 12 minutes

Servings: 3

Ingredients:

- 4 haddock fillets, 5 ounces each, boneless
- 2 tablespoons of coconut oil, melted
- 1 cup of coconut, shredded and unsweetened
- ¼ cup of hazelnuts, ground
- Salt to taste

Directions:

1. Preheat your oven to 400°F.
2. Line a baking sheet with parchment paper.
3. Keep it on the side.
4. Pat fish fillets with a paper towel and season with salt.
5. Take a bowl and stir in hazelnuts and shredded coconut.
6. Drag fish fillets through the coconut mix until both sides are coated well.
7. Transfer to a baking sheet.
8. Brush with coconut oil.
9. Bake for about 12 minutes until flaky.
10. Serve and enjoy!

Nutrition:

Calories: 299

Fat: 24g

Carbohydrates: 1g

Protein: 20g

Vegetable Rice Casserole

Preparation Time: 10 minutes
Cooking Time: 50 minutes
Servings: 4
Ingredients:

- 1 teaspoon of olive oil
- ½ small sweet onion, chopped
- ½ teaspoon of minced garlic
- ½ cup of chopped red bell pepper
- ¼ cup of grated carrot
- 1 cup of white basmati rice
- 2 cups of water
- ¼ cup of grated Parmesan cheese
- Freshly ground black pepper

Directions:

1. Preheat the oven to 350°F.
2. In a medium skillet over medium-high heat, heat the olive oil.
3. Add the onion and garlic, and sauté until softened, about 3 minutes.
4. Transfer the vegetables to a 9-by-9-inch baking sheet, and stir in the rice and water.
5. Cover the dish and bake until the liquid is absorbed 35 to 40 minutes.
6. Sprinkle the cheese on top and bake an additional 5 minutes to melt.
7. Season the casserole with pepper, and serve.

Substitution tip: Not surprisingly, the cheesy topping on this casserole elevates it to a truly sublime experience. You can also try feta, Cheddar cheese, and goat cheese for different tastes and textures.

Nutrition:
Calories: 224
Total fat: 3g
Saturated fat: 1g
Cholesterol: 6mg
Sodium: 105mg
Carbohydrates: 41g
Fiber: 2g
Phosphorus: 118mg
Potassium: 176mg
Protein: 6g

Vegetable Confetti Relish

Preparation Time: 25 minutes

Cooking Time: 15 minutes

Servings: 1

Ingredients:

- ½ red bell pepper
- ½ green pepper, boiled and chopped
- 4 scallions, thinly sliced
- ½ tsp. of ground cumin
- 3 tbsp. of vegetable oil
- 1 ½ tbsp. of white wine vinegar
- Black pepper to taste

Directions:

1. Join all fixings and blend well.
2. Chill in the fridge.
3. You can include a large portion of slashed jalapeno pepper for an increasingly fiery blend

Nutrition:

Calories: 230

Fat: 25g

Fiber: 3g

Carbs: 24g

Protein: 43g

Braised Cabbage

Preparation Time: 10 minutes

Cooking Time: 29 minutes

Servings: 4

Ingredients:

- 1½ tsp. of olive oil
- 2 minced garlic cloves
- 1 thinly sliced onion
- 3 cups of chopped green cabbage
- 1 cup of low- sodium vegetable broth
- Freshly ground black pepper, to taste

Directions:

1. In a large skillet, heat oil on medium-high heat.
2. Add garlic and sauté for about 1 minute.
3. Add onion and sauté for about 4–5 minutes.
4. Add cabbage and sauté for about 3–4 minutes.
5. Stir in broth and black pepper and immediately reduce the heat to low.
6. Cook, covered for about 20 minutes.
7. Serve warm.

Nutrition:

Calories: 45

Fat: 1.8g

Carbs: 6.6g

Protein: 1.1g

Fiber: 1.9g

Potassium: 136mg

Sodium: 46mg

Raw Vegetables. Chopped Salad

Preparation Time: 15 minutes

Cooking Time: 0 minutes

Servings: 1

Ingredients:

- Chopped raw veggie salad
- 1 orange pepper (minced)
- 1 yellow pepper (small cut)
- 5–8 radishes (halve and cut into thin slices) (about 3/4 cup)
- Small head of broccoli (minced) (about 2 cups)
- 1 seedless cucumber (small cut) (about 2 cups)
- 1 cup of halved red seedless grapes
- 2–3 tablespoons of chopped fresh dill
- 1/4 cup of chopped fresh parsley
- 1/4 cup of raw peeled sunflower seeds
- 1/8 cup of raw hemp hearts (peeled hemp seeds)
- Oil-free dressing
- Garlic clove (chopped)
- 1 tablespoon of red wine vinegar
- 1 tablespoon of apple cider vinegar
- 1 lemon juice
- 1 tbsp. of Dijon-senf
- 1 tbsp. of pure maple syrup
- 1/8 tsp. of pepper (or to taste)

Directions:

1. Whisk the ingredients—Chopped raw veggie salad, 1 orange pepper, yellow pepper, radishes, small head of broccoli, seedless cucumber, halved red seedless grapes, chopped fresh dill, chopped fresh parsley, raw peeled sunflower seeds, raw hemp hearts, garlic clove, red wine vinegar, apple cider vinegar, lemon, Dijonsenf, pure maple syrup, pepper.
2. Combine all the salad ingredients in a large bowl.
3. Pour the dressing over the chopped vegetables and wrap well.
4. Cover and then refrigerate it for an hour or two and toss the salad once or twice during this time to coat evenly.
5. Enjoy!

Nutrition:

Calories: 111

Total Fat: 2g

Saturated Fat: 1g

Cholesterol: 10mg

Sodium: 58mg

Carbohydrates: 19g

Sugar: 18g

Calcium: 15g

Broccoli Soup, Green Leaves, and Beans

Preparation Time: 10 minutes

Cooking Time: 40 minutes

Servings: 2

Ingredients:

- 1 tablespoon of olive oil
- 1/2 medium-size onion, cut into large pieces
- 3 cloves of garlic in pieces
- 1 medium-size broccoli head in pieces
- 6 cups of water
- 3 large fleas of green leaves kale.
- 1 fist of coriander leaves and stems
- 11/2 cups of white beans cooked beans
- Freshly ground black pepper
- 2-3 tablespoons of fresh chopped dill
- Lemon juice to serve

Directions:

1. Place a large pot and a lid over medium heat and add the tablespoon of olive oil, onion, garlic. Leave for 5-7 minutes or until the onion is transparent.
2. Add the broccoli and leave for about five minutes or until they change color and start to brown slightly.
3. Add water. Cover and let it begin to boil over low heat.
4. When the broccoli is soft, add the coriander leaves and stems, the dill (if you are going to use it), and the beans.
5. Blend very carefully with a food processor or in the blender. Add black pepper.
6. Before serving, squeeze the juice of a lemon.
7. You can put lemons on the table so that everyone can put more to their liking.

Nutrition:

Calories: 34

Carbohydrate: 6.6g

Fiber: 2.6g

Sugar: 1.7g

Fat: 0.4g

Vegan Vegetable Mini Tortillas

Preparation Time: 10 minutes

Cooking Time: 40 minutes

Servings: 5

Ingredients:

- 1 zucchini
- 1 onion
- 2 carrots
- Pinch of pepper
- 1 teaspoon of Parsley
- 3 small potatoes
- 1 tablespoon of olive oil
- Pinch of comino
- 3 tablespoon of chickpea flour

Directions:

1. Peel potatoes, onions, and carrots. Wash the zucchini and cut all the vegetables into as small as possible (in brunoise).
2. In a pan, fry all the vegetables with a little oil until they are very soft. Comino, pepper, and a few sprigs of chopped parsley and leave over medium heat.
3. We undo the chickpea flour in a little water. It has to be a texture like a beaten egg, so we will be adding the water little by little until it is almost liquid. We add it to the pan of the vegetables and, without stopping to stir, until it is fully integrated. There will be a paste that can be worked with your hands.
4. When the mixture has cooled a little, and we can work by hand, we flour our hands and make balls as twice the size of a meatball. Then we flatten them a bit to give them a hamburger shape, and we put them on the griddle with a drop of oil on both sides.
5. And ready! The vegan vegetable omelets are ready to serve.

Nutrition:

Calories: 196.09

Carbohydrates: 25.4g

Proteins: 6.92g

Vegetarian Recipe

Preparation Time: 10 minutes

Cooking Time: 8 minutes

Servings: 1

Ingredients:

- 1 cup of green beans
- 2 carrots
- Sweet corn
- Cooked rice
- 1 teaspoon of mustard
- A little honey
- Olive oil
- A handful of cooked chickpeas
- 3-4 chopped pistachios

Directions:

1. You have to mix some green beans and some boiled or steamed carrots, along with sweet corn and cooked rice.
2. To dress it, mix a teaspoon of mustard with a little honey and olive oil. And if you want to turn it into a complete and balanced single dish, you can add a handful of cooked chickpeas and three or four chopped pistachios. Besides being delicious, this vegetarian recipe is one of the best meals to take to work.

Nutrition:

Calories: 111

Total Fat: 2g

Saturated Fat: 1g

Cholesterol: 10mg

Sodium: 58mg

Carbohydrates: 19g

Fiber: 0g

Sugar: 18g

Calcium: 15g

White Bean Veggie Burgers

Preparation Time: 10 minutes
Cooking Time: 15 minutes
Servings: 4
Ingredients:

- 1 cup of canned white beans, drained and rinsed
- 1 cup of cooked white rice
- 1 teaspoon of garlic powder
- 2 teaspoons of dried thyme
- ½ teaspoon of ground chipotle pepper
- ½ sweet onion, finely chopped
- ½ cup of fresh or frozen corn
- ½ cup of red bell pepper, finely chopped
- Juice of 1 lemon
- 1/3cup of all-purpose flour
- 1 large egg
- Freshly ground black pepper
- 2 teaspoons of extra-virgin olive oil

Directions:

1. In a large bowl, mash the beans with a potato masher, leaving a few whole beans as desired. Add the rice, garlic powder, thyme, chipotle pepper, onion, corn, bell pepper, lemon, flour, and egg, and mix well to blend. Season with pepper.
2. Using your hands, form the mixture into four patties. Set your oil on in a skillet on medium heat. Cook the burgers for 5 minutes, until browned on one side, flip, and cook the other side for an additional 5 minutes.

Nutrition:
Calories: 305
Fat: 4g
Carbs: 57g
Protein: 11g
Phosphorus: 181mg
Potassium: 515mg
Sodium: 281mg

Spicy Tofu and Broccoli Stir-Fry

Preparation Time: 15 minutes

Cooking Time: 15 minutes

Servings: 4

Ingredients:

For the sauce:

- 3 garlic cloves
- 2-inch piece of ginger, peeled
- 2 tablespoons of honey
- ¼ cup of rice wine vinegar
- 2 tablespoons of extra-virgin olive oil

For the stir-fry:

- 1 (14-ounce) package of extra-firm tofu
- 1 cup of long-grain white rice
- 2 tablespoons of extra-virgin olive oil
- 2 cups of chopped broccoli
- 1 cup of shredded carrots
- 3 scallions, finely chopped

Directions:

To make the sauce:

1. Combine the garlic, ginger, honey, vinegar, and olive oil in a food processor, and purée until smooth.

To make the stir-fry:

2. Cut the tofu into small cubes, and press the excess moisture from the tofu using paper towels, repeating several times until dry. In a medium pot, cook the rice according to package directions.
3. Set your oil on in a skillet on medium heat. Add the tofu to the pan in a single layer. Carefully add ¼ of the sauce to the pan and continue to cook, flipping the tofu only once or twice every 4 minutes, until it is well browned. With a slotted spoon, transfer the tofu to a plate lined with paper towels to drain.
4. Add the broccoli to the pan. Cook, covered, often stirring, until fork-tender, about 5 minutes. Add the carrots and continue to cook for an additional 3 minutes, until

softened. Add the remaining sauce to the vegetables, return the tofu to the pan, and stir to mix. Garnish with scallions and serve over rice.

Nutrition:

Calories: 410

Fat: 18g

Carbs: 51g

Protein: 13g

Phosphorus: 222mg

Potassium: 487mg

Sodium: 51mg